PLANT-BASED RECIPES FOR WEIGHT LOSS AND DIABETES MANAGEMENT

Delicious Recipes for Weight Loss & Diabetes Wellness

Isabella Adams

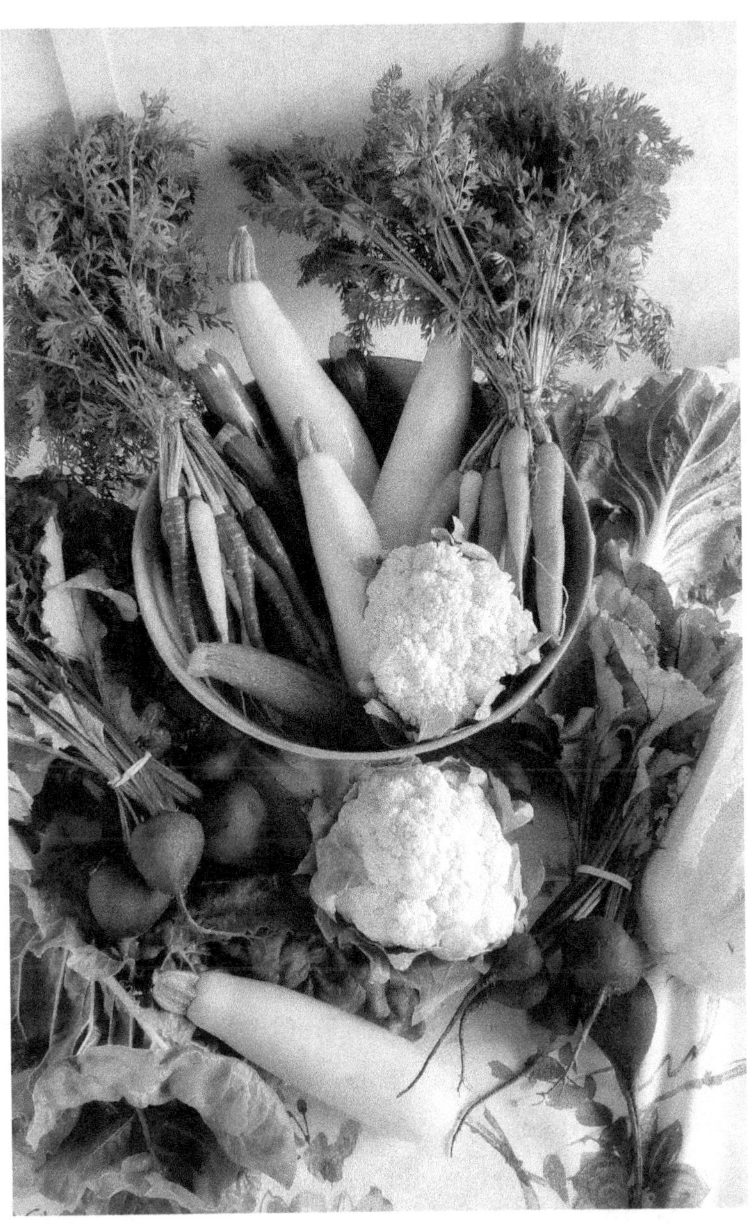

TABLE OF CONTENTS

Chapter 5: Snacks and Appetizers 86

Chapter 6: Desserts 106

INTRODUCTION

Plant-based diets are no longer just a niche trend; they're blossoming into a mainstream movement, driven by both health and ethical concerns. But with so many variations and conflicting information, navigating this world can be daunting. Let's peel back the layers and explore the essence of plant-based eating, its potential benefits for weight management and diabetes control, and the unique considerations to keep in mind.

A Spectrum of Plant-Based Plates: Understanding the Varieties

First, it's crucial to understand that "plant-based" isn't a singular concept. It encompasses a spectrum of dietary approaches, each with varying degrees of animal product inclusion:

- **Vegetarian**: Eliminates meat and poultry, but may include eggs and dairy.

- **Vegan**: Excludes all animal products, including eggs, dairy, and honey.
- **Flexitarian**: Primarily plant-based, but allows occasional animal products for flexibility.
- **Pescatarian**: Primarily plant-based, but includes fish and seafood.

The specific type of plant-based diet you choose depends on your individual preferences, health goals, and ethical considerations.

Weight Management: Can Plants Help Shed Pounds?

The answer is a resounding yes, but it's not just about calorie counting. Plant-based diets tend to be:

- **Lower in calories and saturated fat:** This can lead to a natural calorie deficit, promoting weight loss.
- **Higher in fiber**: Fiber keeps you feeling fuller for longer, reducing cravings and overeating.
- **Rich in water-dense fruits and vegetables:**These contribute to satiety and overall lower calorie intake.

However, simply replacing meat with processed plant-based alternatives won't guarantee weight loss. Focusing on whole, unprocessed plant foods like fruits, vegetables, legumes, and whole grains is key.

Taming the Blood Sugar Beast: Plant-Based Eating and Diabetes

For individuals with type 2 diabetes, plant-based diets offer a powerful tool for managing blood sugar levels:

- **Improved insulin sensitivity:** Plant-based diets are often lower in saturated fat and refined carbohydrates, which can contribute to insulin resistance.
- **Increased fiber intake:** Fiber slows down the absorption of sugar, leading to more stable blood sugar levels.
- **Rich in antioxidants and anti-inflammatory compounds:** These can help protect against diabetes-related complications.

Research consistently shows that plant-based diets can significantly improve blood sugar control, reduce medication needs, and even reverse some aspects of type 2 diabetes.

Beyond Weight and Diabetes: A Holistic Approach

While weight management and diabetes control are significant benefits, the advantages of plant-based eating extend far beyond:

- Reduced risk of heart disease, certain cancers, and other chronic illnesses.
- Improved gut health and microbiome diversity.
- Lower environmental impact and more sustainable food choices.

Remember, embarking on a plant-based journey is a personal decision. With mindful planning and delicious exploration, you can unlock the potential of a plant-based lifestyle for a healthier, happier you.

Bonus Tip: Don't be intimidated! Start small by incorporating more plant-based meals into your week, explore new recipes, and discover the vibrant world of plant-based cuisine. Remember, every step towards a plant-filled future is a step towards a healthier you and a healthier planet.

Chapter 1: 30 Day Meal Plan

Week 1:

Day 1:

- Breakfast: Avocado and Spinach Breakfast Wrap
- Lunch: Lentil and Vegetable Stew
- Dinner: Eggplant and Lentil Lasagna
- Snack: Guacamole with Veggie Sticks
- Dessert: Chocolate Avocado Mousse

Day 2:

- Breakfast: Quinoa and Berry Breakfast Bowl
- Lunch: Quinoa Salad with Roasted Vegetables
- Dinner: Portobello Mushroom Steaks with Garlic Mashed Cauliflower
- Snack: Roasted Red Pepper Hummus with Pita Chips
- Dessert: Vegan Berry Parfait

Day 3:

- Breakfast: Sweet Potato and Black Bean Breakfast Hash

- Lunch: Chickpea and Spinach Curry
- Dinner: Butternut Squash and Sage Risotto
- Snack: Edamame and Sesame Seed Snack
- Dessert: Coconut and Almond Bliss Balls

Day 4:

- Breakfast: Chia Seed Pudding with Fresh Fruits
- Lunch: Grilled Portobello Mushroom Burger
- Dinner: Stuffed Bell Peppers with Quinoa and Black Beans
- Snack: Baked Sweet Potato Fries with Avocado Dip
- Dessert: Baked Apple with Cinnamon and Walnuts

Day 5:

- Breakfast: Oatmeal Pancakes with Maple Syrup
- Lunch: Mediterranean Chickpea Wrap
- Dinner: Cabbage Rolls with Spiced Lentils
- Snack: Spicy Kale Chips
- Dessert: Banana Ice Cream with Nut Toppings

Day 6:

- Breakfast: Blueberry Almond Smoothie Bowl

- Lunch: Spaghetti Squash Primavera
- Dinner: Vegan Creamy Tomato and Basil Pasta
- Snack: Vegan Spinach and Artichoke Dip
- Dessert: Vegan Chocolate Chip Cookies

Day 7:

- Breakfast: Vegan Tofu Scramble with Vegetables
- Lunch: Cauliflower and Chickpea Tacos
- Dinner: Cauliflower and Chickpea Curry
- Snack: Cucumber and Tomato Bruschetta
- Dessert: Chia Seed and Berry Pudding

Week 2:

Day 8:

- Breakfast: Whole Grain Toast with Smashed Avocado
- Lunch: Sweet Potato and Kale Buddha Bowl
- Dinner: Sweet Potato Gnocchi with Sage Butter
- Snack: Mixed Berry Fruit Salsa with Cinnamon Chips
- Dessert: Pumpkin Spice Energy Bites

Day 9:

- Breakfast: Mango and Coconut Overnight Oats
- Lunch: Zucchini Noodles with Pesto
- Dinner: Ratatouille with Polenta
- Snack: Stuffed Mushrooms with Quinoa and Spinach
- Dessert: Avocado and Lime Sorbet

Day 10:

- Breakfast: Mediterranean Chickpea Breakfast Skillet
- Lunch: Thai-Inspired Peanut Tofu Stir-Fry
- Dinner: Wild Rice and Mushroom Stuffed Acorn Squash
- Snack: Avocado and Black Bean Salsa
- Dessert: Almond and Raspberry Thumbprint Cookies

Day 11:

- Breakfast: Berry Quinoa Muffins
- Lunch: Black Bean and Corn Stuffed Peppers
- Dinner: Vegan Chili with Kidney Beans and Corn
- Snack: Roasted Chickpeas with Paprika
- Dessert: Mango and Coconut Chia Seed Popsicles

Day 12:

- Breakfast: Green Smoothie with Kale and Pineapple
- Lunch: Hummus and Veggie Wrap
- Dinner: Mediterranean Stuffed Bell Peppers
- Snack: Vegan Spring Rolls with Peanut Dipping Sauce
- Dessert: Blueberry and Almond Crumble

Day 13:

- Breakfast: Banana Walnut Breakfast Cookies
- Lunch: Brown Rice and Vegetable Sushi Rolls
- Dinner: Spinach and Artichoke-Stuffed Portobello Mushrooms
- Snack: Almond and Cranberry Energy Bites
- Dessert: Pistachio and Cranberry Dark Chocolate Bark

Day 14:

- Breakfast: Spinach and Mushroom Vegan Omelette
- Lunch: Quinoa and Black Bean Burrito Bowl
- Dinner: Lentil and Vegetable Shepherd's Pie
- Snack: Caprese Skewers with Balsamic Glaze

- Dessert: Vegan Lemon Bars

Week 3:

Day 15:

- Breakfast: Papaya and Lime Breakfast Sorbet
- Lunch: Roasted Vegetable and Quinoa Stuffed Acorn Squash
- Dinner: Thai Green Curry with Tofu and Vegetables
- Snack: Watermelon and Mint Gazpacho
- Dessert: Quinoa and Date Energy Bars

Day 16:

- Breakfast: Avocado and Spinach Breakfast Wrap
- Lunch: Lentil and Vegetable Stew
- Dinner: Eggplant and Lentil Lasagna
- Snack: Guacamole with Veggie Sticks
- Dessert: Chocolate Avocado Mousse

Day 17:

- Breakfast: Quinoa and Berry Breakfast Bowl
- Lunch: Quinoa Salad with Roasted Vegetables

- Dinner: Portobello Mushroom Steaks with Garlic Mashed Cauliflower
- Snack: Roasted Red Pepper Hummus with Pita Chips
- Dessert: Vegan Berry Parfait

Day 18:

- Breakfast: Sweet Potato and Black Bean Breakfast Hash
- Lunch: Chickpea and Spinach Curry
- Dinner: Butternut Squash and Sage Risotto
- Snack: Edamame and Sesame Seed Snack
- Dessert: Coconut and Almond Bliss Balls

Day 19:

- Breakfast: Chia Seed Pudding with Fresh Fruits
- Lunch: Grilled Portobello Mushroom Burger
- Dinner: Stuffed Bell Peppers with Quinoa and Black Beans
- Snack: Baked Sweet Potato Fries with Avocado Dip
- Dessert: Baked Apple with Cinnamon and Walnuts

Day 20:

- Breakfast: Oatmeal Pancakes with Maple Syrup
- Lunch: Mediterranean Chickpea Wrap
- Dinner: Cabbage Rolls with Spiced Lentils
- Snack: Spicy Kale Chips
- Dessert: Banana Ice Cream with Nut Toppings

Day 21:

- Breakfast: Blueberry Almond Smoothie Bowl
- Lunch: Spaghetti Squash Primavera
- Dinner: Vegan Creamy Tomato and Basil Pasta
- Snack: Vegan Spinach and Artichoke Dip
- Dessert: Vegan Chocolate Chip Cookies

Week 4:

Day 22:

- Breakfast: Vegan Tofu Scramble with Vegetables
- Lunch: Cauliflower and Chickpea Tacos
- Dinner: Cauliflower and Chickpea Curry
- Snack: Cucumber and Tomato Bruschetta
- Dessert: Chia Seed and Berry Pudding

Day 23:

- Breakfast: Whole Grain Toast with Smashed Avocado
- Lunch: Sweet Potato and Kale Buddha Bowl
- Dinner: Sweet Potato Gnocchi with Sage Butter
- Snack: Mixed Berry Fruit Salsa with Cinnamon Chips
- Dessert: Pumpkin Spice Energy Bites

Day 24:

- Breakfast: Mango and Coconut Overnight Oats
- Lunch: Zucchini Noodles with Pesto
- Dinner: Ratatouille with Polenta
- Snack: Stuffed Mushrooms with Quinoa and Spinach
- Dessert: Avocado and Lime Sorbet

Day 25:

- Breakfast: Mediterranean Chickpea Breakfast Skillet
- Lunch: Thai-Inspired Peanut Tofu Stir-Fry
- Dinner: Wild Rice and Mushroom Stuffed Acorn Squash
- Snack: Avocado and Black Bean Salsa

- Dessert: Almond and Raspberry Thumbprint Cookies

Day 26:

- Breakfast: Berry Quinoa Muffins
- Lunch: Black Bean and Corn Stuffed Peppers
- Dinner: Vegan Chili with Kidney Beans and Corn
- Snack: Roasted Chickpeas with Paprika
- Dessert: Mango and Coconut Chia Seed Popsicles

Day 27:

- Breakfast: Green Smoothie with Kale and Pineapple
- Lunch: Hummus and Veggie Wrap
- Dinner: Mediterranean Stuffed Bell Peppers
- Snack: Vegan Spring Rolls with Peanut Dipping Sauce
- Dessert: Blueberry and Almond Crumble

Day 28:

- Breakfast: Banana Walnut Breakfast Cookies
- Lunch: Brown Rice and Vegetable Sushi Rolls

- Dinner: Spinach and Artichoke-Stuffed Portobello Mushrooms
- Snack: Almond and Cranberry Energy Bites
- Dessert: Pistachio and Cranberry Dark Chocolate Bark

Day 29:

- Breakfast: Spinach and Mushroom Vegan Omelette
- Lunch: Quinoa and Black Bean Burrito Bowl
- Dinner: Lentil and Vegetable Shepherd's Pie
- Snack: Caprese Skewers with Balsamic Glaze
- Dessert: Vegan Lemon Bars

Day 30:

- Breakfast: Papaya and Lime Breakfast Sorbet
- Lunch: Roasted Vegetable and Quinoa Stuffed Acorn Squash
- Dinner: Thai Green Curry with Tofu and Vegetables
- Snack: Watermelon and Mint Gazpacho
- Dessert: Quinoa and Date Energy Bars

Chapter 2: Breakfast Recipes

In this Chapter, we dive into the realm of breakfast, presenting unique and delectable recipes designed to kickstart your day with a burst of flavor and nutrition. Each recipe brings together vibrant ingredients and thoughtful combinations, ensuring a delightful experience for your taste buds and a nutritious boost for your body.

Avocado and Spinach Breakfast Wrap

Ingredients:

- 1 whole-grain tortilla
- 1 ripe avocado, sliced
- Handful of fresh spinach leaves
- Cherry tomatoes, sliced
- 1 tablespoon hummus
- Salt and pepper to taste

Instructions:

1. Lay the tortilla flat and spread hummus evenly.

2. Arrange avocado slices, spinach, and tomatoes.

3. Season with salt and pepper.

4. Roll the tortilla tightly.

5. Slice in half and serve.

Nutrition Information:

- Calories: 300

- Protein: 7g

- Carbohydrates: 30g

- Fat: 18g

- Fiber: 9g

- Sugar: 2g

- Portion Size: 1 wrap

Quinoa and Berry Breakfast Bowl

Ingredients:

- 1 cup cooked quinoa

- Mixed berries (strawberries, blueberries, raspberries)

- 1 tablespoon almond butter

- 1 tablespoon chia seeds

- Drizzle of maple syrup

Instructions:

1. In a bowl, layer cooked quinoa.
2. Top with mixed berries and chia seeds.
3. Drizzle almond butter and maple syrup.
4. Gently mix and enjoy.

Nutrition Information:

- Calories: 350
- Protein: 10g
- Carbohydrates: 45g
- Fat: 15g
- Fiber: 8g
- Sugar: 10g
- Portion Size: 1 bowl

Sweet Potato and Black Bean Breakfast Hash

Ingredients:

- 1 sweet potato, diced
- 1 can black beans, drained and rinsed
- Red bell pepper, chopped

- Onion, diced
- 1 teaspoon cumin
- Salt and pepper to taste

Instructions:

1. Sauté sweet potatoes, black beans, bell pepper, and onion.
2. Add cumin, salt, and pepper.
3. Cook until sweet potatoes are tender.
4. Serve warm.

Nutrition Information:

- Calories: 280
- Protein: 8g
- Carbohydrates: 50g
- Fat: 2g
- Fiber: 12g
- Sugar: 6g
- Portion Size: 1 serving

Chia Seed Pudding with Fresh Fruits

Ingredients:

- 2 tablespoons chia seeds
- 1 cup almond milk
- Mixed fresh fruits (berries, kiwi, mango)
- 1 tablespoon honey or agave syrup
- 1 teaspoon vanilla extract

Instructions:

1. Mix chia seeds, almond milk, honey or agave, and vanilla.
2. Refrigerate overnight or until pudding consistency.
3. Layer with fresh fruits before serving.

Nutrition Information:

- Calories: 220
- Protein: 5g
- Carbohydrates: 35g
- Fat: 8g
- Fiber: 10g
- Sugar: 15g
- Portion Size: 1 serving

Oatmeal Pancakes with Maple Syrup

Ingredients:

- 1 cup rolled oats
- 1 ripe banana, mashed
- 1 cup almond milk
- 1 teaspoon baking powder
- Maple syrup for drizzling

Instructions:

1. Blend oats, banana, almond milk, and baking powder.
2. Pour batter onto a heated skillet.
3. Cook until bubbles appear, flip, and cook the other side.
4. Drizzle with maple syrup before serving.

Nutrition Information:

- Calories: 280
- Protein: 7g
- Carbohydrates: 55g
- Fat: 4g
- Fiber: 8g

- Sugar: 12g
- Portion Size: 2 pancakes

Blueberry Almond Smoothie Bowl

Ingredients:

- 1 cup frozen blueberries
- 1 banana
- 1 cup almond milk
- 1 tablespoon almond butter
- Toppings: sliced almonds, fresh blueberries

Instructions:

1. Blend frozen blueberries, banana, almond milk, and almond butter.
2. Pour into a bowl and add toppings.

Nutrition Information:

- Calories: 250
- Protein: 6g
- Carbohydrates: 40g
- Fat: 10g
- Fiber: 9g

- Sugar: 18g
- Portion Size: 1 bowl

Vegan Tofu Scramble with Vegetables

Ingredients:

- 1 block firm tofu, crumbled
- Bell peppers, onions, and spinach
- 1 tablespoon nutritional yeast
- 1 teaspoon turmeric
- Salt and pepper to taste

Instructions:

1. Sauté tofu, bell peppers, onions, and spinach.
2. Add nutritional yeast, turmeric, salt, and pepper.
3. Cook until veggies are tender.

Nutrition Information:

- Calories: 220
- Protein: 15g
- Carbohydrates: 10g

- Fat: 14g

- Fiber: 4g

- Sugar: 2g

- Portion Size: 1 serving

Whole Grain Toast with Smashed Avocado

Ingredients:

- 2 slices whole-grain bread

- 1 ripe avocado

- Cherry tomatoes, sliced

- Red pepper flakes (optional)

- Lemon juice

- Salt and pepper to taste

Instructions:

1. Toast the bread slices.

2. Smash avocado on the toast.

3. Top with sliced cherry tomatoes.

4. Drizzle with lemon juice, and season with red pepper flakes, salt, and pepper.

Nutrition Information:

- Calories: 280
- Protein: 8g
- Carbohydrates: 30g
- Fat: 15g
- Fiber: 12g
- Sugar: 2g
- Portion Size: 1 serving

Mango and Coconut Overnight Oats

Ingredients:

- 1/2 cup rolled oats
- 1/2 cup almond milk
- 1/2 cup diced mango
- 2 tablespoons shredded coconut
- 1 tablespoon chia seeds

Instructions:

1. Mix oats, almond milk, mango, coconut, and chia seeds.
2. Refrigerate overnight.
3. Stir before serving.

Nutrition Information:

- Calories: 320
- Protein: 8g
- Carbohydrates: 45g
- Fat: 12g
- Fiber: 9g
- Sugar: 15g
- Portion Size: 1 serving

Mediterranean Chickpea Breakfast Skillet

Ingredients:

- 1 can chickpeas, drained and rinsed
- Cherry tomatoes, halved
- Spinach leaves
- Red onion, finely chopped
- 1 clove garlic, minced
- 1 teaspoon cumin
- 1 tablespoon olive oil
- Salt and pepper to taste

Instructions:

1. Sauté red onion and garlic in olive oil until fragrant.
2. Add chickpeas, cherry tomatoes, and spinach.
3. Season with cumin, salt, and pepper.
4. Cook until spinach wilts.

Nutrition Information:

- Calories: 280
- Protein: 10g
- Carbohydrates: 35g
- Fat: 12g
- Fiber: 10g
- Sugar: 5g
- Portion Size: 1 serving

Berry Quinoa Muffins

Ingredients:

- 1 cup cooked quinoa
- 1 cup mixed berries (blueberries, raspberries)
- 1 cup oat flour
- 1/2 cup almond milk
- 1/4 cup maple syrup

- 1 teaspoon baking powder
- 1/2 teaspoon vanilla extract

Instructions:

1. Preheat oven to 350°F (175°C).
2. Mix quinoa, berries, oat flour, almond milk, maple syrup, baking powder, and vanilla.
3. Spoon batter into muffin cups.
4. Bake for 20-25 minutes.

Nutrition Information:

- Calories: 180
- Protein: 5g
- Carbohydrates: 30g
- Fat: 5g
- Fiber: 4g
- Sugar: 10g
- Portion Size: 1 muffin

Green Smoothie with Kale and Pineapple

Ingredients:

- 1 cup kale leaves, stems removed
- 1 cup pineapple chunks
- 1/2 banana
- 1/2 cup coconut water
- Ice cubes

Instructions:

1. Blend kale, pineapple, banana, and coconut water until smooth.
2. Add ice cubes and blend again.
3. Pour into a glass and enjoy.

Nutrition Information:

- Calories: 120
- Protein: 3g
- Carbohydrates: 30g
- Fat: 1g
- Fiber: 5g
- Sugar: 15g

- Portion Size: 1 glass

Banana Walnut Breakfast Cookies

Ingredients:

- 2 ripe bananas, mashed
- 1 cup rolled oats
- 1/2 cup chopped walnuts
- 1/4 cup almond butter
- 1 teaspoon cinnamon
- 1/2 teaspoon vanilla extract

Instructions:

1. Preheat oven to 350°F (175°C).
2. In a bowl, combine mashed bananas, oats, walnuts, almond butter, cinnamon, and vanilla.
3. Spoon onto a baking sheet and flatten each cookie.
4. Bake for 12-15 minutes.

Nutrition Information:

- Calories: 160
- Protein: 4g
- Carbohydrates: 20g

- Fat: 8g

- Fiber: 3g

- Sugar: 7g

- Portion Size: 2 cookies

Spinach and Mushroom Vegan Omelette

Ingredients:

- 1 cup chickpea flour

- 1 1/4 cups water

- Handful of fresh spinach

- Mushrooms, sliced

- 1/4 cup diced tomatoes

- 1/4 cup red bell pepper, chopped

- Salt and pepper to taste

Instructions:

1. Whisk chickpea flour and water until smooth.

2. Sauté spinach, mushrooms, tomatoes, and bell pepper.

3. Pour the chickpea batter over the veggies.

4. Cook until the edges lift, then flip and cook the other side.

Nutrition Information:

- Calories: 200
- Protein: 10g
- Carbohydrates: 25g
- Fat: 7g
- Fiber: 6g
- Sugar: 5g
- Portion Size: 1 serving

Papaya and Lime Breakfast Sorbet

Ingredients:

- 2 cups ripe papaya, diced
- Juice of 1 lime
- 1 tablespoon agave syrup
- Mint leaves for garnish

Instructions:

1. Blend papaya, lime juice, and agave syrup until smooth.

2. Pour into a shallow dish and freeze.

3. Scoop into bowls, garnish with mint, and serve.

Nutrition Information:

- Calories: 120
- Protein: 1g
- Carbohydrates: 30g
- Fat: 0.5g
- Fiber: 3g
- Sugar: 20g
- Portion Size: 1 bowl

Chapter 3: Lunch Recipes

These lunch recipes are not just meals; they are a celebration of vibrant ingredients, diverse textures, and nourishing goodness. From hearty stews to tantalizing wraps, each dish is crafted to satisfy your palate while promoting a healthy lifestyle.

Lentil and Vegetable Stew

Ingredients:

- 1 cup green lentils, rinsed
- 2 carrots, diced
- 1 onion, chopped
- 3 cloves garlic, minced
- 1 zucchini, sliced
- 1 can diced tomatoes
- 4 cups vegetable broth
- 1 teaspoon cumin
- 1 teaspoon paprika
- Salt and pepper to taste

Instructions:

1. In a large pot, sauté onions and garlic until fragrant.
2. Add lentils, carrots, zucchini, tomatoes, and vegetable broth.
3. Season with cumin, paprika, salt, and pepper.
4. Simmer for 25-30 minutes until lentils are tender.
5. Serve hot.

Nutrition Information:

- Calories: 250
- Protein: 15g
- Carbohydrates: 45g
- Fat: 2g
- Fiber: 12g
- Sugar: 5g
- Portion Size: 1 cup

Quinoa Salad with Roasted Vegetables

Ingredients:

- 1 cup quinoa, cooked

- 1 bell pepper, sliced

- 1 zucchini, diced

- 1 cup cherry tomatoes, halved

- 1 red onion, thinly sliced

- 2 tablespoons olive oil

- 1 teaspoon dried oregano

- Salt and pepper to taste

Instructions:

1. Preheat oven to 400°F (200°C).

2. Toss vegetables in olive oil, oregano, salt, and pepper.

3. Roast for 20-25 minutes until veggies are tender.

4. Mix with cooked quinoa.

5. Drizzle with extra olive oil if desired.

Nutrition Information:

- Calories: 320

- Protein: 8g

- Carbohydrates: 55g

- Fat: 10g

- Fiber: 9g

- Sugar: 5g
- Portion Size: 1.5 cups

Chickpea and Spinach Curry

Ingredients:

- 1 can chickpeas, drained and rinsed
- 2 cups spinach leaves
- 1 onion, finely chopped
- 2 tomatoes, diced
- 3 cloves garlic, minced
- 1 tablespoon curry powder
- 1 teaspoon turmeric
- 1 can coconut milk
- Salt and pepper to taste

Instructions:

1. In a pan, sauté onions and garlic until translucent.
2. Add chickpeas, tomatoes, curry powder, and turmeric. Cook for 5 minutes.
3. Pour in coconut milk and simmer for another 10 minutes.
4. Add spinach, cook until wilted.

5. Season with salt and pepper.

Nutrition Information:

- Calories: 280
- Protein: 10g
- Carbohydrates: 30g
- Fat: 15g
- Fiber: 8g
- Sugar: 5g
- Portion Size: 1.5 cups

Grilled Portobello Mushroom Burger

Ingredients:

- 4 large Portobello mushrooms
- 4 whole grain burger buns
- 1 red onion, sliced
- 4 lettuce leaves
- 4 tomato slices
- 1/4 cup balsamic vinegar
- 2 tablespoons olive oil
- Salt and pepper to taste

Instructions:

1. Mix balsamic vinegar, olive oil, salt, and pepper in a bowl.

2. Brush mushrooms with the mixture and grill for 5-7 minutes on each side.

3. Assemble burgers with lettuce, tomato, and onion.

Nutrition Information:

- Calories: 220
- Protein: 8g
- Carbohydrates: 35g
- Fat: 6g
- Fiber: 7g
- Sugar: 8g
- Portion Size: 1 burger

Mediterranean Chickpea Wrap

Ingredients:

- 1 can chickpeas, mashed
- 4 whole wheat wraps
- 1 cucumber, sliced
- 1 cup cherry tomatoes, halved

- 1/2 cup Kalamata olives, sliced
- 1/4 cup feta cheese, crumbled
- Tzatziki sauce for drizzling

Instructions:

1. Spread mashed chickpeas on wraps.
2. Add cucumber, tomatoes, olives, and feta.
3. Drizzle with tzatziki sauce.
4. Roll tightly and cut in half.

Nutrition Information:

- Calories: 320
- Protein: 12g
- Carbohydrates: 45g
- Fat: 10g
- Fiber: 10g
- Sugar: 5g
- Portion Size: 1 wrap

Spaghetti Squash Primavera

Ingredients:

- 1 medium spaghetti squash, halved

- 2 cups cherry tomatoes, halved
- 1 bell pepper, sliced
- 1 zucchini, diced
- 3 cloves garlic, minced
- 2 tablespoons olive oil
- 1 teaspoon dried basil
- Salt and pepper to taste

Instructions:

1. Preheat oven to 400°F (200°C).
2. Roast spaghetti squash for 40-45 minutes.
3. In a pan, sauté garlic, add tomatoes, bell pepper, and zucchini.
4. Toss in cooked spaghetti squash strands.
5. Season with basil, salt, and pepper.

Nutrition Information:

- Calories: 220
- Protein: 5g
- Carbohydrates: 35g
- Fat: 8g
- Fiber: 10g

- Sugar: 10g
- Portion Size: 1.5 cups

Cauliflower and Chickpea Tacos

Ingredients:

- 1 head cauliflower, chopped
- 1 can chickpeas, drained and rinsed
- 1 tablespoon taco seasoning
- 8 small corn tortillas
- 1 cup shredded purple cabbage
- 1 avocado, sliced
- Lime wedges for serving

Instructions:

1. Roast cauliflower and chickpeas with taco seasoning.
2. Warm tortillas and fill with cauliflower, chickpeas, cabbage, and avocado.
3. Squeeze lime over the top.

Nutrition Information:

- Calories: 280
- Protein: 9g

- Carbohydrates: 45g

- Fat: 10g

- Fiber: 12g

- Sugar: 5g

- Portion Size: 2 tacos

Sweet Potato and Kale Buddha Bowl

Ingredients:

- 2 sweet potatoes, cubed

- 2 cups kale, chopped

- 1 cup quinoa, cooked

- 1/4 cup tahini

- 2 tablespoons lemon juice

- 1 tablespoon soy sauce

- 1 tablespoon maple syrup

Instructions:

1. Roast sweet potatoes until golden.

2. Massage kale with lemon juice.

3. Assemble bowls with quinoa, sweet potatoes, and kale.

4. Drizzle with a sauce made from tahini, soy sauce, and maple syrup.

Nutrition Information:

- Calories: 350
- Protein: 12g
- Carbohydrates: 55g
- Fat: 10g
- Fiber: 10g
- Sugar: 8g
- Portion Size: 2 cups

Zucchini Noodles with Pesto

Ingredients:

- 4 medium zucchinis, spiralized
- 1 cup cherry tomatoes, halved
- 1/2 cup pine nuts, toasted
- 2 cups fresh basil leaves
- 1/2 cup nutritional yeast
- 2 cloves garlic
- 1/2 cup olive oil
- Salt and pepper to taste

Instructions:

1. Spiralize zucchinis into noodles.
2. In a food processor, blend basil, pine nuts, nutritional yeast, and garlic.
3. Gradually add olive oil until a smooth pesto forms.
4. Toss zucchini noodles with cherry tomatoes and pesto.
5. Season with salt and pepper.

Nutrition Information:

- Calories: 280
- Protein: 8g
- Carbohydrates: 15g
- Fat: 20g
- Fiber: 5g
- Sugar: 5g
- Portion Size: 1.5 cups

Thai-Inspired Peanut Tofu Stir-Fry

Ingredients:

- 1 block firm tofu, cubed
- 2 cups broccoli florets

- 1 bell pepper, sliced
- 1 carrot, julienned
- 2 tablespoons soy sauce
- 3 tablespoons peanut butter
- 1 tablespoon maple syrup
- 1 teaspoon ginger, grated
- 1 clove garlic, minced

Instructions:

1. Sauté tofu until golden.
2. Add broccoli, bell pepper, and carrot.
3. In a bowl, mix soy sauce, peanut butter, maple syrup, ginger, and garlic.
4. Pour over tofu and vegetables, stir until well-coated.

Nutrition Information:

- Calories: 320
- Protein: 15g
- Carbohydrates: 25g
- Fat: 18g
- Fiber: 8g
- Sugar: 10g

- Portion Size: 1.5 cups

Black Bean and Corn Stuffed Peppers

Ingredients:

- 4 bell peppers, halved
- 1 can black beans, drained and rinsed
- 1 cup corn kernels
- 1 cup cooked quinoa
- 1 cup salsa
- 1 teaspoon cumin
- 1/2 teaspoon chili powder
- 1/2 cup vegan cheese (optional)

Instructions:

1. Preheat oven to 375°F (190°C).
2. Mix black beans, corn, quinoa, salsa, cumin, and chili powder.
3. Stuff peppers with the mixture.
4. Top with vegan cheese if desired.
5. Bake for 25-30 minutes.

Nutrition Information:

- Calories: 280
- Protein: 12g
- Carbohydrates: 45g
- Fat: 5g
- Fiber: 10g
- Sugar: 5g
- Portion Size: 1.5 peppers

Hummus and Veggie Wrap

Ingredients:

- 4 whole wheat wraps
- 1 cup hummus
- 1 cucumber, thinly sliced
- 1 bell pepper, julienned
- 1 carrot, shredded
- 1 cup mixed greens
- Salt and pepper to taste

Instructions:

1. Spread hummus evenly on each wrap.

2. Layer with cucumber, bell pepper, carrot, and mixed greens.

3. Season with salt and pepper.

4. Roll tightly and slice in half.

Nutrition Information:

- Calories: 300

- Protein: 10g

- Carbohydrates: 40g

- Fat: 12g

- Fiber: 10g

- Sugar: 5g

- Portion Size: 1 wrap

Brown Rice and Vegetable Sushi Rolls

Ingredients:

- 2 cups brown rice, cooked

- 4 nori sheets

- 1 cucumber, julienned

- 1 carrot, julienned

- 1 avocado, sliced
- Soy sauce for dipping
- Pickled ginger and wasabi for serving

Instructions:

1. Place nori sheet on a bamboo sushi rolling mat.
2. Spread a layer of brown rice.
3. Add cucumber, carrot, and avocado.
4. Roll tightly and slice into bite-sized pieces.
5. Serve with soy sauce, pickled ginger, and wasabi.

Nutrition Information:

- Calories: 250
- Protein: 8g
- Carbohydrates: 45g
- Fat: 5g
- Fiber: 8g
- Sugar: 2g
- Portion Size: 6 pieces

Quinoa and Black Bean Burrito Bowl

Ingredients:

- 1 cup quinoa, cooked
- 1 can black beans, drained and rinsed
- 1 cup corn kernels
- 1 avocado, diced
- 1 tomato, diced
- 1/4 cup fresh cilantro, chopped
- Lime wedges for serving
- Salt and pepper to taste

Instructions:

1. Arrange quinoa, black beans, corn, avocado, and tomato in a bowl.
2. Sprinkle with cilantro.
3. Season with salt and pepper.
4. Squeeze lime over the top.

Nutrition Information:

- Calories: 320
- Protein: 12g
- Carbohydrates: 50g

- Fat: 10g

- Fiber: 12g

- Sugar: 5g

- Portion Size: 2 cups

Roasted Vegetable and Quinoa Stuffed Acorn Squash

Ingredients:

- 2 acorn squashes, halved

- 1 cup quinoa, cooked

- 1 zucchini, diced

- 1 red onion, diced

- 1 bell pepper, diced

- 2 tablespoons olive oil

- 1 teaspoon dried thyme

- Salt and pepper to taste

Instructions:

1. Preheat oven to 375°F (190°C).

2. Place acorn squash halves on a baking sheet.

3. In a bowl, mix quinoa, zucchini, red onion, bell pepper, olive oil, thyme, salt, and pepper.
4. Stuff each squash half with the quinoa mixture.
5. Bake for 30-35 minutes until squash is tender.

Nutrition Information:

- Calories: 280
- Protein: 8g
- Carbohydrates: 45g
- Fat: 10g
- Fiber: 10g
- Sugar: 5g
- Portion Size: 1 stuffed squash half

Chapter 4: Dinner Recipes

These dishes are not only a treat for your taste buds but are also designed to bring wholesome satisfaction to your dinner table. From hearty lasagna to flavorful stuffed peppers, each recipe is a celebration of plant-based goodness. Let's embark on a culinary journey that caters to both your taste and well-being.

Eggplant and Lentil Lasagna

Ingredients:

- 2 medium-sized eggplants, sliced
- 1 cup dry green or brown lentils
- 2 cups tomato sauce
- 1 cup spinach, chopped
- 1 teaspoon dried oregano
- 1 teaspoon garlic powder
- Salt and pepper to taste
- 2 cups vegan mozzarella cheese, shredded

Instructions:

1. Cook lentils according to package instructions.
2. Preheat the oven to 375°F (190°C).
3. In a baking dish, layer sliced eggplants, cooked lentils, tomato sauce, chopped spinach, oregano, and garlic powder.
4. Repeat the layers and top with vegan mozzarella.
5. Bake for 30-35 minutes until the top is golden brown.
6. Allow it to cool for a few minutes before serving.

Nutrition Information:

- Calories: 320
- Protein: 15g
- Carbohydrates: 45g
- Fat: 12g
- Fiber: 12g
- Sugar: 8g
- Portion Size: 1 slice

Portobello Mushroom Steaks with Garlic Mashed Cauliflower

Ingredients:

- 4 large Portobello mushrooms
- 1 tablespoon balsamic vinegar
- 2 tablespoons olive oil
- 4 cloves garlic, minced
- 1 head cauliflower, chopped
- Salt and pepper to taste
- Fresh parsley for garnish

Instructions:

1. Preheat the grill or grill pan.
2. Mix balsamic vinegar, olive oil, and minced garlic. Brush over Portobello mushrooms.
3. Grill mushrooms for 5-7 minutes on each side.
4. Boil cauliflower until tender, then mash with garlic, salt, and pepper.
5. Serve Portobello steaks on a bed of garlic mashed cauliflower.
6. Garnish with fresh parsley.

Nutrition Information:

- Calories: 180
- Protein: 8g
- Carbohydrates: 20g
- Fat: 10g
- Fiber: 7g
- Sugar: 6g
- Portion Size: 1 mushroom steak with cauliflower

Butternut Squash and Sage Risotto

Ingredients:

- 1 cup Arborio rice
- 3 cups butternut squash, diced
- 1 onion, finely chopped
- 4 cups vegetable broth, heated
- 1/2 cup dry white wine
- 2 tablespoons nutritional yeast
- 1 tablespoon fresh sage, chopped
- Salt and pepper to taste
- 2 tablespoons vegan butter

Instructions:

1. Sauté onions in vegan butter until translucent.
2. Add Arborio rice and cook until lightly toasted.
3. Pour in white wine and stir until absorbed.
4. Add butternut squash and gradually ladle in warm vegetable broth.
5. Stir continuously until rice is creamy and cooked.
6. Stir in nutritional yeast, sage, salt, and pepper.
7. Serve hot.

Nutrition Information:

- Calories: 280
- Protein: 5g
- Carbohydrates: 60g
- Fat: 4g
- Fiber: 6g
- Sugar: 4g
- Portion Size: 1 cup

Stuffed Bell Peppers with Quinoa and Black Beans

Ingredients:

- 4 large bell peppers, halved
- 1 cup quinoa, cooked
- 1 can black beans, drained and rinsed
- 1 cup corn kernels
- 1 cup tomatoes, diced
- 1 teaspoon cumin
- 1 teaspoon chili powder
- Salt and pepper to taste
- Fresh cilantro for garnish

Instructions:

1. Preheat the oven to 375°F (190°C).
2. Mix quinoa, black beans, corn, tomatoes, cumin, chili powder, salt, and pepper.
3. Stuff bell peppers with the quinoa mixture.
4. Bake for 25-30 minutes until peppers are tender.
5. Garnish with fresh cilantro before serving.

Nutrition Information:

- Calories: 220
- Protein: 8g
- Carbohydrates: 40g
- Fat: 2g
- Fiber: 8g
- Sugar: 6g
- Portion Size: 2 stuffed pepper halves

Cabbage Rolls with Spiced Lentils

Ingredients:

- 1 head cabbage
- 1 cup dry red lentils
- 1 onion, finely chopped
- 2 cloves garlic, minced
- 1 can tomato sauce
- 1 teaspoon smoked paprika
- 1 teaspoon cayenne pepper
- Salt and pepper to taste
- 1 cup vegetable broth

Instructions:

1. Preheat the oven to 375°F (190°C).
2. Boil cabbage leaves until soft, then set aside.
3. Cook lentils with onion, garlic, smoked paprika, cayenne pepper, salt, and pepper.
4. Place a spoonful of lentil mixture on each cabbage leaf and roll tightly.
5. Arrange rolls in a baking dish, cover with tomato sauce and vegetable broth.
6. Bake for 25-30 minutes.

Nutrition Information:

- Calories: 250
- Protein: 15g
- Carbohydrates: 45g
- Fat: 2g
- Fiber: 12g
- Sugar: 8g
- Portion Size: 2 rolls

Vegan Creamy Tomato and Basil Pasta

Ingredients:

- 8 oz whole wheat or gluten-free pasta
- 2 cups cherry tomatoes, halved
- 1 can coconut milk
- 1/4 cup nutritional yeast
- 1/4 cup fresh basil, chopped
- 3 cloves garlic, minced
- Salt and pepper to taste
- Red pepper flakes for optional spice

Instructions:

1. Cook pasta according to package instructions.
2. In a pan, combine coconut milk, nutritional yeast, garlic, salt, and pepper.
3. Add cherry tomatoes and cook until softened.
4. Toss cooked pasta in the creamy tomato sauce.
5. Garnish with fresh basil and red pepper flakes.

Nutrition Information:

- Calories: 400

- Protein: 10g
- Carbohydrates: 60g
- Fat: 16g
- Fiber: 8g
- Sugar: 4g
- Portion Size: 1.5 cups

Cauliflower and Chickpea Curry

Ingredients:

- 1 medium cauliflower, cut into florets
- 1 can chickpeas, drained and rinsed
- 1 onion, finely chopped
- 3 tomatoes, diced
- 1 can coconut milk
- 2 tablespoons curry powder
- 1 teaspoon turmeric
- Salt and pepper to taste
- Fresh cilantro for garnish

Instructions:

1. Sauté onion until translucent in a large pot.

2. Add cauliflower, chickpeas, tomatoes, curry powder, turmeric, salt, and pepper.

3. Pour in coconut milk and simmer until cauliflower is tender.

4. Garnish with fresh cilantro before serving.

5. Serve over rice or quinoa.

Nutrition Information:

- Calories: 320
- Protein: 12g
- Carbohydrates: 45g
- Fat: 14g
- Fiber: 10g
- Sugar: 8g
- Portion Size: 1.5 cups

Sweet Potato Gnocchi with Sage Butter

Ingredients:

- 2 large sweet potatoes, peeled and diced
- 2 cups whole wheat flour or gluten-free flour

- 1/4 cup vegan butter
- 1 tablespoon fresh sage, chopped
- Salt and pepper to taste
- 1/4 cup nutritional yeast (optional)

Instructions:

1. Boil sweet potatoes until fork-tender; mash thoroughly.
2. Mix mashed sweet potatoes with flour until a dough forms.
3. Roll dough into ropes and cut into bite-sized pieces.
4. Boil gnocchi until they float to the surface.
5. In a pan, melt vegan butter, add sage, salt, and pepper.
6. Toss cooked gnocchi in the sage butter.
7. Sprinkle with nutritional yeast if desired.

Nutrition Information:

- Calories: 280
- Protein: 8g
- Carbohydrates: 50g
- Fat: 6g

- Fiber: 8g

- Sugar: 4g

- Portion Size: 1 cup

Ratatouille with Polenta

Ingredients:

- 1 eggplant, sliced

- 2 zucchinis, sliced

- 2 bell peppers, sliced

- 3 tomatoes, sliced

- 1 onion, diced

- 3 cloves garlic, minced

- 2 tablespoons tomato paste

- 1 teaspoon dried thyme

- Salt and pepper to taste

- 1 cup polenta, cooked

Instructions:

1. Preheat the oven to 375°F (190°C).

2. In a baking dish, layer eggplant, zucchini, bell peppers, tomatoes, onion, and garlic.

3. Mix tomato paste, thyme, salt, and pepper; spread over the vegetables.

4. Bake for 40-45 minutes until vegetables are tender.

5. Serve over a bed of cooked polenta.

Nutrition Information:

- Calories: 250

- Protein: 6g

- Carbohydrates: 55g

- Fat: 2g

- Fiber: 12g

- Sugar: 10g

- Portion Size: 1.5 cups with polenta

Wild Rice and Mushroom Stuffed Acorn Squash

Ingredients:

- 2 acorn squash, halved and seeds removed

- 1 cup wild rice, cooked

- 1 cup mushrooms, diced

- 1 onion, finely chopped

- 2 cloves garlic, minced
- 1/4 cup fresh parsley, chopped
- 2 tablespoons olive oil
- Salt and pepper to taste
- 1/4 cup toasted pecans, chopped

Instructions:

1. Preheat the oven to 400°F (200°C).
2. Place acorn squash halves on a baking sheet, cut side down, and bake for 30 minutes.
3. Sauté onion and garlic in olive oil until softened.
4. Add mushrooms and cook until browned.
5. Mix cooked wild rice, mushroom mixture, parsley, salt, and pepper.
6. Stuff the baked acorn squash halves with the rice mixture.
7. Top with toasted pecans before serving.

Nutrition Information:

- Calories: 320
- Protein: 8g
- Carbohydrates: 60g

- Fat: 10g
- Fiber: 10g
- Sugar: 6g
- Portion Size: 1 stuffed acorn squash half

Vegan Chili with Kidney Beans and Corn

Ingredients:

- 2 cans kidney beans, drained and rinsed
- 1 cup corn kernels
- 1 onion, diced
- 3 cloves garlic, minced
- 1 can diced tomatoes
- 1 can tomato sauce
- 2 tablespoons chili powder
- 1 teaspoon cumin
- Salt and pepper to taste
- 1 cup vegetable broth

Instructions:

1. In a large pot, sauté onions and garlic until softened.

2. Add kidney beans, corn, diced tomatoes, tomato sauce, chili powder, cumin, salt, and pepper.

3. Pour in vegetable broth and simmer for 20-25 minutes.

4. Adjust seasoning to taste.

5. Serve hot.

Nutrition Information:

- Calories: 280
- Protein: 12g
- Carbohydrates: 50g
- Fat: 2g
- Fiber: 12g
- Sugar: 8g
- Portion Size: 1.5 cups

Mediterranean Stuffed Bell Peppers

Ingredients:

- 4 large bell peppers, halved
- 1 cup cooked quinoa
- 1 cup cherry tomatoes, halved
- 1 cucumber, diced

- 1/2 cup Kalamata olives, chopped
- 1/4 cup red onion, finely chopped
- 1/4 cup fresh parsley, chopped
- 2 tablespoons olive oil
- Juice of 1 lemon
- Salt and pepper to taste

Instructions:

1. Preheat the oven to 375°F (190°C).
2. Mix quinoa, cherry tomatoes, cucumber, olives, red onion, parsley, olive oil, lemon juice, salt, and pepper.
3. Stuff bell peppers with the Mediterranean quinoa mixture.
4. Bake for 25-30 minutes.
5. Serve warm.

Nutrition Information:

- Calories: 240
- Protein: 6g
- Carbohydrates: 40g
- Fat: 8g

- Fiber: 8g

- Sugar: 6g

- Portion Size: 2 stuffed pepper halves

Spinach and Artichoke-Stuffed Portobello Mushrooms

Ingredients:

- 4 large Portobello mushrooms

- 2 cups fresh spinach, chopped

- 1 can artichoke hearts, drained and chopped

- 1/2 cup vegan cream cheese

- 2 cloves garlic, minced

- 1/4 cup nutritional yeast

- Salt and pepper to taste

- 2 tablespoons olive oil

Instructions:

1. Preheat the oven to 375°F (190°C).

2. Remove stems from Portobello mushrooms and place them on a baking sheet.

3. In a bowl, mix spinach, artichoke hearts, vegan cream cheese, garlic, nutritional yeast, salt, and pepper.

4. Stuff the Portobello mushrooms with the spinach and artichoke mixture.

5. Drizzle olive oil over the mushrooms.

6. Bake for 20-25 minutes until mushrooms are tender.

Nutrition Information:

- Calories: 220

- Protein: 8g

- Carbohydrates: 20g

- Fat: 14g

- Fiber: 6g

- Sugar: 4g

- Portion Size: 1 stuffed mushroom

Lentil and Vegetable Shepherd's Pie

Ingredients:

- 2 cups green or brown lentils, cooked

- 1 onion, diced

- 2 carrots, diced

- 1 cup peas
- 1 cup corn kernels
- 3 cloves garlic, minced
- 1 cup vegetable broth
- 2 tablespoons tomato paste
- 1 teaspoon thyme
- Mashed potatoes for topping
- Salt and pepper to taste

Instructions:

1. Preheat the oven to 400°F (200°C).
2. In a pan, sauté onions, carrots, peas, corn, and garlic until softened.
3. Add cooked lentils, vegetable broth, tomato paste, thyme, salt, and pepper.
4. Transfer the lentil and vegetable mixture to a baking dish.
5. Top with mashed potatoes.
6. Bake for 25-30 minutes until the top is golden brown.

Nutrition Information:

- Calories: 300

- Protein: 12g

- Carbohydrates: 55g

- Fat: 2g

- Fiber: 12g

- Sugar: 6g

- Portion Size: 1 cup

Thai Green Curry with Tofu and Vegetables

Ingredients:

- 1 block extra-firm tofu, pressed and cubed

- 2 cups mixed vegetables (bell peppers, broccoli, carrots)

- 1 can coconut milk

- 2 tablespoons Thai green curry paste

- 1 tablespoon soy sauce

- 1 tablespoon maple syrup

- 1 tablespoon lime juice

- Fresh cilantro for garnish

- Cooked brown rice for serving

Instructions:

1. In a pan, sauté tofu until golden brown; set aside.

2. In the same pan, stir-fry mixed vegetables until slightly tender.

3. Add coconut milk, Thai green curry paste, soy sauce, maple syrup, and lime juice.

4. Bring to a simmer, then add tofu back to the pan.

5. Simmer for 10-15 minutes until vegetables are cooked.

6. Garnish with fresh cilantro.

7. Serve over cooked brown rice.

Nutrition Information:

- Calories: 350
- Protein: 15g
- Carbohydrates: 40g
- Fat: 18g
- Fiber: 8g
- Sugar: 10g
- Portion Size: 1.5 cups with rice

Chapter 5: Snacks and Appetizers

These recipes are crafted to tantalize your taste buds while keeping health in mind. From vibrant guacamole to refreshing watermelon and mint gazpacho, each recipe offers a burst of flavors that make snacking a delightful experience.

Guacamole with Veggie Sticks

Ingredients:

- 3 ripe avocados
- 1 medium-sized tomato, diced
- 1/4 cup red onion, finely chopped
- 1 clove garlic, minced
- 1 lime, juiced
- Salt and pepper to taste

Instructions:

1. In a bowl, mash the avocados with a fork.
2. Add diced tomatoes, chopped red onion, minced garlic, and lime juice. Mix well.

3. Season with salt and pepper to taste.

4. Serve with an assortment of colorful veggie sticks.

Nutrition Information:

- Calories: 120

- Protein: 2g

- Carbohydrates: 7g

- Fat: 10g

- Fiber: 5g

- Sugar: 1g

- Portion Size: 1/4 cup guacamole with veggie sticks

Roasted Red Pepper Hummus with Pita Chips

Ingredients:

- 1 can (15 oz) chickpeas, drained and rinsed

- 1/3 cup tahini

- 1/4 cup lemon juice

- 1/4 cup roasted red peppers

- 2 cloves garlic

- 2 tablespoons olive oil

- Salt to taste

Instructions:

1. Combine chickpeas, tahini, lemon juice, roasted red peppers, and garlic in a food processor.
2. Blend until smooth, adding olive oil gradually. Season with salt.
3. Serve with homemade or store-bought whole wheat pita chips.

Nutrition Information:

- Calories: 160
- Protein: 4g
- Carbohydrates: 12g
- Fat: 11g
- Fiber: 3g
- Sugar: 1g
- Portion Size: 1/4 cup hummus with pita chips

Edamame and Sesame Seed Snack

Ingredients:

- 2 cups edamame (frozen, thawed)

- 1 tablespoon sesame oil

- 1 tablespoon soy sauce

- 1 tablespoon sesame seeds (toasted)

Instructions:

1. Steam or boil edamame until tender. Drain and pat dry.

2. In a bowl, toss edamame with sesame oil, soy sauce, and toasted sesame seeds.

Nutrition Information:

- Calories: 120

- Protein: 11g

- Carbohydrates: 7g

- Fat: 7g

- Fiber: 4g

- Sugar: 2g

- Portion Size: 1/2 cup edamame and sesame seed mix

Baked Sweet Potato Fries with Avocado Dip

Ingredients:

- 2 large sweet potatoes, cut into fries
- 2 tablespoons olive oil
- 1 teaspoon paprika
- 1/2 teaspoon garlic powder
- Salt and pepper to taste

Avocado Dip:

- 2 ripe avocados
- 1/4 cup plain vegan yogurt
- 1 tablespoon lime juice
- Salt and pepper to taste

Instructions:

1. Preheat the oven to 425°F (220°C).
2. Toss sweet potato fries with olive oil, paprika, garlic powder, salt, and pepper.
3. Arrange fries on a baking sheet and bake for 25-30 minutes or until crispy.

4. In a blender, combine avocados, vegan yogurt, lime juice, salt, and pepper. Blend until smooth.

5. Serve the baked sweet potato fries with the avocado dip.

Nutrition Information:

- Calories: 180

- Protein: 3g

- Carbohydrates: 20g

- Fat: 10g

- Fiber: 5g

- Sugar: 2g

- Portion Size: 1 cup sweet potato fries with 2 tablespoons avocado dip

Spicy Kale Chips

Ingredients:

- 1 bunch kale, stems removed and torn into pieces

- 1 tablespoon olive oil

- 1 teaspoon chili powder

- 1/2 teaspoon cayenne pepper

- Salt to taste

Instructions:

1. Preheat the oven to 300°F (150°C).

2. In a bowl, toss kale with olive oil, chili powder, cayenne pepper, and salt.

3. Spread kale on a baking sheet and bake for 15-20 minutes until crispy.

Nutrition Information:

- Calories: 50

- Protein: 2g

- Carbohydrates: 6g

- Fat: 3g

- Fiber: 2g

- Sugar: 1g

- Portion Size: 1 cup spicy kale chips

Vegan Spinach and Artichoke Dip

Ingredients:

- 1 cup raw cashews, soaked

- 1 cup frozen spinach, thawed and drained

- 1 can (14 oz) artichoke hearts, chopped

- 2 cloves garlic, minced

- 1/4 cup nutritional yeast
- 1 tablespoon lemon juice
- Salt and pepper to taste

Instructions:

1. In a food processor, blend soaked cashews, thawed spinach, chopped artichoke hearts, minced garlic, nutritional yeast, and lemon juice until smooth.
2. Season with salt and pepper to taste.
3. Serve as a dip with sliced veggies or whole-grain crackers.

Nutrition Information:

- Calories: 120
- Protein: 5g
- Carbohydrates: 10g
- Fat: 8g
- Fiber: 3g
- Sugar: 1g
- Portion Size: 1/4 cup spinach and artichoke dip

Cucumber and Tomato Bruschetta

Ingredients:

- 2 cups cherry tomatoes, halved
- 1 cucumber, diced
- 1/4 cup red onion, finely chopped
- 2 tablespoons fresh basil, chopped
- 2 tablespoons balsamic vinegar
- 1 tablespoon olive oil
- Salt and pepper to taste

Instructions:

1. In a bowl, combine cherry tomatoes, cucumber, red onion, and fresh basil.
2. Drizzle with balsamic vinegar and olive oil. Season with salt and pepper.
3. Toss gently and let it marinate for 15 minutes.
4. Serve on whole grain toast or crackers.

Nutrition Information:

- Calories: 70
- Protein: 1g
- Carbohydrates: 8g

- Fat: 4g

- Fiber: 2g

- Sugar: 4g

- Portion Size: 1/2 cup bruschetta mix

Mixed Berry Fruit Salsa with Cinnamon Chips

Ingredients:

- 1 cup strawberries, diced

- 1/2 cup blueberries

- 1/2 cup raspberries

- 1 tablespoon fresh mint, chopped

- 1 tablespoon maple syrup

- 4 whole wheat tortillas

- 1 tablespoon coconut oil, melted

- 1 teaspoon cinnamon

Instructions:

1. In a bowl, combine strawberries, blueberries, raspberries, mint, and maple syrup.

2. Preheat the oven to 350°F (175°C).

3. Brush tortillas with melted coconut oil, sprinkle with cinnamon, and cut into triangles.

4. Bake tortilla triangles for 8-10 minutes until crispy.

5. Serve the mixed berry salsa with cinnamon chips.

Nutrition Information:

- Calories: 120

- Protein: 2g

- Carbohydrates: 20g

- Fat: 4g

- Fiber: 5g

- Sugar: 7g

- Portion Size: 1/2 cup salsa with 4 cinnamon chips

Stuffed Mushrooms with Quinoa and Spinach

Ingredients:

- 12 large mushrooms, stems removed

- 1 cup cooked quinoa

- 1 cup baby spinach, chopped

- 1/4 cup sun-dried tomatoes, diced

- 2 cloves garlic, minced

- 1/4 cup nutritional yeast

- Salt and pepper to taste

Instructions:

1. Preheat the oven to 375°F (190°C).

2. In a bowl, mix cooked quinoa, chopped spinach, sun-dried tomatoes, minced garlic, nutritional yeast, salt, and pepper.

3. Stuff mushrooms with the quinoa mixture and bake for 15-20 minutes until mushrooms are tender.

Nutrition Information:

- Calories: 80

- Protein: 4g

- Carbohydrates: 15g

- Fat: 1g

- Fiber: 3g

- Sugar: 2g

- Portion Size: 2 stuffed mushrooms

Avocado and Black Bean Salsa

Ingredients:

- 1 can (15 oz) black beans, drained and rinsed
- 1 avocado, diced
- 1 cup corn kernels (fresh or frozen)
- 1/4 cup red onion, finely chopped
- 1 jalapeño, seeded and minced
- 2 tablespoons fresh cilantro, chopped
- 1 lime, juiced
- Salt and pepper to taste

Instructions:

1. In a bowl, combine black beans, diced avocado, corn, red onion, jalapeño, and cilantro.
2. Squeeze lime juice over the mixture and toss gently.
3. Season with salt and pepper to taste.
4. Serve with whole-grain tortilla chips.

Nutrition Information:

- Calories: 120
- Protein: 5g
- Carbohydrates: 20g

- Fat: 4g

- Fiber: 7g

- Sugar: 2g

- Portion Size: 1/2 cup salsa with tortilla chips

Roasted Chickpeas with Paprika

Ingredients:

- 2 cans (15 oz each) chickpeas, drained and rinsed

- 2 tablespoons olive oil

- 1 teaspoon smoked paprika

- 1/2 teaspoon garlic powder

- 1/2 teaspoon cumin

- Salt to taste

Instructions:

1. Preheat the oven to 400°F (200°C).

2. Pat chickpeas dry and toss with olive oil, smoked paprika, garlic powder, cumin, and salt.

3. Spread chickpeas on a baking sheet and roast for 30-40 minutes, shaking the pan occasionally.

4. Allow to cool before serving.

Nutrition Information:

- Calories: 150
- Protein: 7g
- Carbohydrates: 19g
- Fat: 6g
- Fiber: 5g
- Sugar: 2g
- Portion Size: 1/2 cup roasted chickpeas

Vegan Spring Rolls with Peanut Dipping Sauce

Ingredients:

For Spring Rolls:

- 10 rice paper wrappers
- 2 cups vermicelli rice noodles, cooked
- 1 cup lettuce, shredded
- 1 cup cucumber, julienned
- 1 cup carrot, julienned
- 1/2 cup fresh mint leaves
- 1/2 cup cilantro leaves

For Peanut Dipping Sauce:

- 1/4 cup creamy peanut butter
- 2 tablespoons soy sauce
- 1 tablespoon maple syrup
- 1 tablespoon lime juice
- 1 teaspoon sriracha (optional)
- Water (for thinning)

Instructions:

For Spring Rolls:

1. Soften rice paper wrappers in warm water according to package instructions.
2. Fill each wrapper with a small portion of rice noodles, lettuce, cucumber, carrot, mint, and cilantro.
3. Roll tightly, tucking in the sides.

For Peanut Dipping Sauce:

1. Whisk together peanut butter, soy sauce, maple syrup, lime juice, and sriracha.
2. Add water gradually until desired consistency is reached.

3. Serve spring rolls with peanut dipping sauce.

Nutrition Information:

- Calories: 180
- Protein: 5g
- Carbohydrates: 30g
- Fat: 6g
- Fiber: 3g
- Sugar: 4g
- Portion Size: 2 spring rolls with dipping sauce

Almond and Cranberry Energy Bites

Ingredients:

- 1 cup rolled oats
- 1/2 cup almond butter
- 1/3 cup honey or maple syrup
- 1/2 cup almonds, chopped
- 1/2 cup dried cranberries
- 1 teaspoon vanilla extract
- Pinch of salt

Instructions:

1. In a bowl, combine rolled oats, almond butter, honey or maple syrup, chopped almonds, dried cranberries, vanilla extract, and a pinch of salt.

2. Mix until well combined.

3. Form mixture into small energy bites and refrigerate for at least 30 minutes.

Nutrition Information:

- Calories: 120
- Protein: 3g
- Carbohydrates: 15g
- Fat: 6g
- Fiber: 2g
- Sugar: 7g
- Portion Size: 2 energy bites

Caprese Skewers with Balsamic Glaze

Ingredients:

- Cherry tomatoes

- Fresh mozzarella balls
- Fresh basil leaves
- Balsamic glaze

Instructions:

1. Thread cherry tomatoes, fresh mozzarella balls, and fresh basil leaves onto skewers.
2. Arrange on a serving platter and drizzle with balsamic glaze.

Nutrition Information:

- Calories: 70
- Protein: 4g
- Carbohydrates: 2g
- Fat: 5g
- Fiber: 1g
- Sugar: 1g
- Portion Size: 3 skewers

Watermelon and Mint Gazpacho

Ingredients:

- 4 cups seedless watermelon, diced

- 1 cucumber, peeled and diced
- 1 red bell pepper, diced
- 1/4 cup red onion, finely chopped
- 2 tablespoons fresh mint, chopped
- 2 tablespoons lime juice
- Salt and pepper to taste

Instructions:

1. In a blender, combine watermelon, cucumber, red bell pepper, red onion, mint, and lime juice.
2. Blend until smooth.
3. Season with salt and pepper to taste.
4. Chill in the refrigerator before serving.

Nutrition Information:

- Calories: 60
- Protein: 1g
- Carbohydrates: 15g
- Fat: 0g
- Fiber: 1g
- Sugar: 10g
- Portion Size: 1 cup gazpacho

Chapter 6: Desserts

In this chapter, we explore unique and scrumptious plant-based desserts that not only satisfy your sweet tooth but also align with your health goals. From creamy mousses to fruity popsicles, these recipes promise a symphony of flavors without the guilt.

Chocolate Avocado Mousse

Ingredients:

- 2 ripe avocados
- 1/4 cup cocoa powder
- 1/4 cup maple syrup
- 1 tsp vanilla extract
- Pinch of salt

Instructions:

1. Blend avocados until smooth.
2. Add cocoa powder, maple syrup, vanilla extract, and a pinch of salt.
3. Blend until creamy and refrigerate.

Nutrition Information:

- Calories: 150
- Protein: 2g
- Carbohydrates: 15g
- Fat: 10g
- Fiber: 6g
- Sugar: 6g
- Portion Size: 1/2 cup

Vegan Berry Parfait

Ingredients:

- 1 cup mixed berries
- 1 cup coconut yogurt
- 1/2 cup granola
- 1 tbsp agave syrup

Instructions:

1. Layer berries, yogurt, and granola in a glass.
2. Repeat layers.
3. Drizzle agave syrup on top.

Nutrition Information:

- Calories: 220
- Protein: 5g
- Carbohydrates: 30g
- Fat: 10g
- Fiber: 8g
- Sugar: 12g
- Portion Size: 1 serving

Coconut and Almond Bliss Balls

Ingredients:

- 1 cup dates, pitted
- 1/2 cup almonds
- 1/4 cup shredded coconut
- 2 tbsp cocoa powder
- 1 tbsp coconut oil

Instructions:

1. Blend dates, almonds, coconut, and cocoa powder.
2. Add coconut oil, blend until sticky.
3. Roll into balls and refrigerate.

Nutrition Information:

- Calories: 120
- Protein: 3g
- Carbohydrates: 15g
- Fat: 7g
- Fiber: 4g
- Sugar: 10g
- Portion Size: 2 balls

Baked Apple with Cinnamon and Walnuts

Ingredients:

- 4 apples, cored
- 1/4 cup chopped walnuts
- 2 tbsp maple syrup
- 1 tsp cinnamon

Instructions:

1. Preheat oven to 375°F (190°C).
2. Mix walnuts, maple syrup, and cinnamon.

3. Stuff apples with the mixture and bake for 20-25 minutes.

Nutrition Information:

- Calories: 180
- Protein: 2g
- Carbohydrates: 30g
- Fat: 8g
- Fiber: 6g
- Sugar: 22g
- Portion Size: 1 apple

Banana Ice Cream with Nut Toppings

Ingredients:

- 4 ripe bananas, frozen
- 1/4 cup chopped mixed nuts
- 1 tbsp coconut flakes

Instructions:

1. Blend frozen bananas until creamy.

2. Top with chopped nuts and coconut flakes.

Nutrition Information:

- Calories: 160
- Protein: 3g
- Carbohydrates: 25g
- Fat: 7g
- Fiber: 4g
- Sugar: 14g
- Portion Size: 1 cup

Vegan Chocolate Chip Cookies

Ingredients:

- 1 cup almond flour
- 1/2 cup coconut sugar
- 1/4 cup coconut oil
- 1 tsp vanilla extract
- 1/2 cup dairy-free chocolate chips

Instructions:

1. Mix almond flour, coconut sugar, coconut oil, and vanilla.

2. Fold in chocolate chips.

3. Form into cookies and bake for 12-15 minutes.

Nutrition Information:

- Calories: 120

- Protein: 2g

- Carbohydrates: 10g

- Fat: 8g

- Fiber: 2g

- Sugar: 6g

- Portion Size: 2 cookies

Chia Seed and Berry Pudding

Ingredients:

- 1/4 cup chia seeds

- 1 cup almond milk

- 1 tbsp maple syrup

- 1 cup mixed berries

Instructions:

1. Mix chia seeds, almond milk, and maple syrup. Refrigerate overnight.

2. Layer chia pudding with mixed berries.

Nutrition Information:

- Calories: 180
- Protein: 4g
- Carbohydrates: 20g
- Fat: 8g
- Fiber: 10g
- Sugar: 8g
- Portion Size: 1 serving

Pumpkin Spice Energy Bites

Ingredients:

- 1 cup rolled oats
- 1/2 cup pumpkin puree
- 1/4 cup almond butter
- 2 tbsp maple syrup
- 1 tsp pumpkin spice

Instructions:

1. Mix oats, pumpkin puree, almond butter, maple syrup, and pumpkin spice.

2. Form into bite-sized balls and refrigerate.

Nutrition Information:

- Calories: 150
- Protein: 5g
- Carbohydrates: 20g
- Fat: 7g
- Fiber: 3g
- Sugar: 6g
- Portion Size: 3 bites

Avocado and Lime Sorbet

Ingredients:

- 2 ripe avocados
- 1/2 cup coconut milk
- 1/4 cup lime juice
- 1/4 cup agave syrup

Instructions:

1. Blend avocados, coconut milk, lime juice, and agave syrup.

2. Freeze in an ice cream maker or a shallow dish.

Nutrition Information:

- Calories: 160
- Protein: 2g
- Carbohydrates: 18g
- Fat: 10g
- Fiber: 5g
- Sugar: 10g
- Portion Size: 1/2 cup

Almond and Raspberry Thumbprint Cookies

Ingredients:

- 1 cup almond flour
- 1/4 cup coconut oil, melted
- 1/4 cup maple syrup
- 1/4 cup raspberry jam

Instructions:

1. Mix almond flour, melted coconut oil, and maple syrup.

2. Form into cookies, make a thumbprint, and add raspberry jam.
3. Bake for 10-12 minutes.

Nutrition Information:

- Calories: 140

- Protein: 3g

- Carbohydrates: 14g

- Fat: 9g

- Fiber: 2g

- Sugar: 8g

- Portion Size: 2 cookies

Mango and Coconut Chia Seed Popsicles

Ingredients:

- 2 cups mango chunks

- 1/2 cup coconut milk

- 2 tbsp chia seeds

- 1 tbsp agave syrup

Instructions:

1. Blend mango chunks and coconut milk.

2. Stir in chia seeds and agave syrup.

3. Pour into popsicle molds and freeze.

Nutrition Information:

- Calories: 120

- Protein: 2g

- Carbohydrates: 18g

- Fat: 5g

- Fiber: 4g

- Sugar: 12g

- Portion Size: 1 popsicle

Blueberry and Almond Crumble

Ingredients:

- 2 cups blueberries

- 1 cup almond flour

- 1/4 cup coconut oil, solid

- 1/4 cup maple syrup

- 1/2 cup rolled oats

Instructions:

1. Mix blueberries with almond flour and maple syrup.

2. Combine solid coconut oil and oats until crumbly.

3. Sprinkle crumble on top and bake for 25-30 minutes.

Nutrition Information:

- Calories: 180

- Protein: 4g

- Carbohydrates: 20g

- Fat: 10g

- Fiber: 5g

- Sugar: 10g

- Portion Size: 1 serving

Pistachio and Cranberry Dark Chocolate Bark

Ingredients:

- 1 cup dark chocolate, melted

- 1/4 cup pistachios, chopped

- 1/4 cup dried cranberries

Instructions:

1. Melt dark chocolate and spread it on a parchment-lined tray.
2. Sprinkle chopped pistachios and dried cranberries on top.
3. Refrigerate until set and break into pieces.

Nutrition Information:

- Calories: 150
- Protein: 2g
- Carbohydrates: 15g
- Fat: 10g
- Fiber: 3g
- Sugar: 10g
- Portion Size: 2 squares

Vegan Lemon Bars

Ingredients:

- 1 cup almond flour
- 1/4 cup coconut oil, melted
- 1/4 cup maple syrup
- 1/2 cup lemon juice

- Zest of one lemon

Instructions:

1. Mix almond flour, melted coconut oil, and maple syrup.
2. Press into a baking dish to form the crust.
3. Mix lemon juice and zest, pour over the crust, and bake for 15-20 minutes.

Nutrition Information:

- Calories: 130
- Protein: 3g
- Carbohydrates: 15g
- Fat: 7g
- Fiber: 2g
- Sugar: 8g
- Portion Size: 1 bar

Quinoa and Date Energy Bars

Ingredients:

- 1 cup cooked quinoa
- 1/2 cup dates, pitted

- 1/4 cup almond butter
- 1/4 cup shredded coconut
- 1 tsp vanilla extract

Instructions:

1. Blend cooked quinoa, dates, almond butter, shredded coconut, and vanilla extract.
2. Press into a pan and refrigerate.
3. Cut into bars before serving.

Nutrition Information:

- Calories: 160
- Protein: 4g
- Carbohydrates: 20g
- Fat: 8g
- Fiber: 3g
- Sugar: 10g
- Portion Size: 1 bar

Chapter 7: Smoothies

These plant-powered concoctions are not just refreshing but are designed to cater to various palates and dietary preferences. Get ready to embark on a journey of flavors with our unique smoothie recipes, each offering a delicious blend of wholesome ingredients to keep you energized throughout the day.

Green Detox Smoothie

Ingredients:

- 1 cup kale leaves, stems removed
- 1/2 cucumber, peeled and sliced
- 1 green apple, cored and chopped
- 1/2 lemon, juiced
- 1 cup coconut water
- Ice cubes (optional)

Instructions:

1. Combine kale, cucumber, green apple, and lemon juice in a blender.

2. Add coconut water and blend until smooth.

3. If desired, add ice cubes and blend again until well combined.

4. Pour into a glass and enjoy the refreshing detox goodness!

Nutrition Information:

- Calories: 120
- Protein: 3g
- Carbohydrates: 25g
- Fat: 1g
- Fiber: 5g
- Sugar: 15g
- Portion Size: 1 serving

Berry Blast Smoothie

Ingredients:

- 1 cup mixed berries (strawberries, blueberries, raspberries)
- 1 banana, peeled and frozen
- 1/2 cup almond milk
- 1 tablespoon chia seeds

- 1 tablespoon honey (optional)

Instructions:

1. Combine mixed berries, frozen banana, almond milk, and chia seeds in a blender.
2. Blend until smooth and creamy.
3. Add honey if additional sweetness is desired.
4. Pour into a glass and savor the burst of berry flavors!

Nutrition Information:

- Calories: 180
- Protein: 4g
- Carbohydrates: 35g
- Fat: 3g
- Fiber: 8g
- Sugar: 18g
- Portion Size: 1 serving

Mango Tango Smoothie

Ingredients:

- 1 cup diced mango
- 1/2 cup pineapple chunks

- 1/2 cup orange juice
- 1/2 cup Greek yogurt (or plant-based yogurt)
- Ice cubes (optional)

Instructions:

1. Combine diced mango, pineapple chunks, orange juice, and Greek yogurt in a blender.
2. Blend until smooth and creamy.
3. Add ice cubes if a colder consistency is preferred.
4. Pour into a glass and indulge in the tropical dance of flavors!

Nutrition Information:

- Calories: 150
- Protein: 6g
- Carbohydrates: 30g
- Fat: 2g
- Fiber: 4g
- Sugar: 22g
- Portion Size: 1 serving

Pineapple Coconut Paradise Smoothie

Ingredients:

- 1 cup pineapple chunks
- 1/2 cup coconut milk
- 1/4 cup shredded coconut
- 1 tablespoon lime juice
- 1 tablespoon agave syrup (optional)
- Ice cubes (optional)

Instructions:

1. Blend pineapple chunks, coconut milk, shredded coconut, and lime juice until smooth.
2. Add agave syrup if additional sweetness is desired.
3. Incorporate ice cubes for a frosty texture.
4. Pour into a glass and transport yourself to a tropical paradise!

Nutrition Information:

- Calories: 160
- Protein: 2.5g
- Carbohydrates: 20g

- Fat: 8g

- Fiber: 3g

- Sugar: 15g

- Portion Size: 1 serving

Spinach and Pineapple Smoothie

Ingredients:

- 2 cups fresh spinach leaves

- 1 cup diced pineapple

- 1 banana, peeled

- 1/2 cup coconut water

- 1 tablespoon flaxseeds

- Ice cubes (optional)

Instructions:

1. Blend spinach, diced pineapple, banana, and coconut water until smooth.

2. Add flaxseeds for an extra nutritional boost.

3. Integrate ice cubes if a colder consistency is preferred.

4. Pour into a glass and relish the green vitality!

Nutrition Information:

- Calories: 130
- Protein: 3.5g
- Carbohydrates: 28g
- Fat: 1.5g
- Fiber: 6g
- Sugar: 15g
- Portion Size: 1 serving

Chocolate Almond Butter Smoothie

Ingredients:

- 1 cup almond milk
- 1 banana, peeled and frozen
- 2 tablespoons almond butter
- 1 tablespoon cocoa powder
- 1 teaspoon maple syrup
- Ice cubes (optional)

Instructions:

1. Blend almond milk, frozen banana, almond butter, cocoa powder, and maple syrup until smooth.
2. Include ice cubes for a thicker texture.

3. Pour into a glass and savor the rich chocolate indulgence!

Nutrition Information:

- Calories: 220
- Protein: 7g
- Carbohydrates: 25g
- Fat: 12g
- Fiber: 5g
- Sugar: 12g
- Portion Size: 1 serving

Citrus Burst Smoothie

Ingredients:

- 1 orange, peeled and segmented
- 1/2 grapefruit, peeled and segmented
- 1 cup pineapple chunks
- 1/2 cup Greek yogurt (or plant-based yogurt)
- 1 tablespoon honey (optional)
- Ice cubes (optional)

Instructions:

1. Blend orange segments, grapefruit segments, pineapple chunks, Greek yogurt, and honey until smooth.
2. Incorporate ice cubes for a refreshing chill.
3. Pour into a glass and enjoy the zesty burst of citrus flavors!

Nutrition Information:

- Calories: 140
- Protein: 5g
- Carbohydrates: 30g
- Fat: 1.5g
- Fiber: 4g
- Sugar: 22g
- Portion Size: 1 serving

Tropical Turmeric Smoothie

Ingredients:

- 1 cup mango chunks
- 1/2 banana, peeled and frozen
- 1/2 teaspoon turmeric powder

- 1/2 cup coconut water

- 1 tablespoon chia seeds

- Ice cubes (optional)

Instructions:

1. Blend mango chunks, frozen banana, turmeric powder, coconut water, and chia seeds until smooth.

2. Add ice cubes for a refreshing twist.

3. Pour into a glass and enjoy the tropical turmeric fusion!

Nutrition Information:

- Calories: 170

- Protein: 4g

- Carbohydrates: 30g

- Fat: 5g

- Fiber: 6g

- Sugar: 18g

- Portion Size: 1 serving

Blueberry Kale Power Smoothie

Ingredients:

- 1 cup blueberries
- 1 cup kale leaves, stems removed
- 1/2 cup plain Greek yogurt (or plant-based yogurt)
- 1 tablespoon almond butter
- 1 tablespoon honey
- Ice cubes (optional)

Instructions:

1. Blend blueberries, kale leaves, Greek yogurt, almond butter, and honey until smooth.
2. Incorporate ice cubes for a chilled texture.
3. Pour into a glass and relish the powerful blend of blueberries and kale!

Nutrition Information:

- Calories: 200
- Protein: 8g
- Carbohydrates: 30g
- Fat: 6g
- Fiber: 5g

- Sugar: 20g
- Portion Size: 1 serving

Peanut Butter Banana Protein Smoothie

Ingredients:

- 1 banana, peeled
- 2 tablespoons peanut butter
- 1 cup almond milk
- 1 scoop plant-based protein powder
- 1 tablespoon flaxseeds
- Ice cubes (optional)

Instructions:

1. Blend banana, peanut butter, almond milk, plant-based protein powder, and flaxseeds until smooth.
2. Include ice cubes for an extra chill.
3. Pour into a glass and enjoy the protein-packed goodness!

Nutrition Information:

- Calories: 250
- Protein: 15g
- Carbohydrates: 20g
- Fat: 12g
- Fiber: 6g
- Sugar: 10g
- Portion Size: 1 serving

Cucumber Mint Cooler Smoothie

Ingredients:

- 1 cucumber, peeled and sliced
- 1/2 cup fresh mint leaves
- 1/2 lime, juiced
- 1 cup coconut water
- 1 tablespoon agave syrup (optional)
- Ice cubes (optional)

Instructions:

1. Blend cucumber slices, fresh mint leaves, lime juice, coconut water, and agave syrup until smooth.
2. Add ice cubes for a cooler sensation.

3. Pour into a glass and savor the refreshing cucumber mint delight!

Nutrition Information:

- Calories: 90
- Protein: 1g
- Carbohydrates: 20g
- Fat: 0.5g
- Fiber: 3g
- Sugar: 12g
- Portion Size: 1 serving

Watermelon Basil Refresher Smoothie

Ingredients:

- 2 cups fresh watermelon, seeded and cubed
- 1/4 cup fresh basil leaves
- 1/2 lemon, juiced
- 1 cup coconut water
- 1 tablespoon honey (optional)
- Ice cubes (optional)

Instructions:

1. Blend watermelon cubes, fresh basil leaves, lemon juice, coconut water, and honey until smooth.
2. Integrate ice cubes for a cool sensation.
3. Pour into a glass and relish the hydrating watermelon basil refresher!

Nutrition Information:

- Calories: 120
- Protein: 2g
- Carbohydrates: 30g
- Fat: 0.5g
- Fiber: 2g
- Sugar: 25g
- Portion Size: 1 serving

Raspberry and Avocado Green Smoothie

Ingredients:

- 1/2 cup fresh or frozen raspberries
- 1/2 avocado, peeled and pitted

- 1 cup spinach leaves
- 1/2 cup almond milk
- 1 tablespoon chia seeds
- Ice cubes (optional)

Instructions:

1. Blend raspberries, avocado, spinach leaves, almond milk, and chia seeds until smooth.
2. Include ice cubes for a chilled consistency.
3. Pour into a glass and enjoy the fusion of raspberry sweetness with creamy avocado!

Nutrition Information:

- Calories: 180
- Protein: 4g
- Carbohydrates: 20g
- Fat: 10g
- Fiber: 8g
- Sugar: 8g
- Portion Size: 1 serving

Pomegranate Berry Antioxidant Smoothie

Ingredients:

- 1/2 cup pomegranate seeds
- 1/2 cup mixed berries (blueberries, strawberries)
- 1/2 cup Greek yogurt (or plant-based yogurt)
- 1 tablespoon honey
- 1/2 cup water
- Ice cubes (optional)

Instructions:

1. Blend pomegranate seeds, mixed berries, Greek yogurt, honey, and water until smooth.
2. Add ice cubes for a refreshing twist.
3. Pour into a glass and indulge in the antioxidant-rich goodness!

Nutrition Information:

- Calories: 150
- Protein: 5g
- Carbohydrates: 25g
- Fat: 2g

- Fiber: 6g

- Sugar: 18g

- Portion Size: 1 serving

Golden Turmeric Latte Smoothie

Ingredients:

- 1 banana, peeled and frozen

- 1/2 teaspoon turmeric powder

- 1/2 teaspoon ginger, grated

- 1 cup almond milk

- 1 tablespoon maple syrup

- Ice cubes (optional)

Instructions:

1. Blend frozen banana, turmeric powder, grated ginger, almond milk, and maple syrup until smooth.

2. Include ice cubes for a colder texture.

3. Pour into a glass and enjoy the warmth of a golden turmeric latte in smoothie form!

Nutrition Information:

- Calories: 170

- Protein: 2g
- Carbohydrates: 35g
- Fat: 3g
- Fiber: 4g
- Sugar: 22g
- Portion Size: 1 serving

CONCLUSION

As we conclude this journey through "Plant-Based Recipes for Weight Loss and Diabetes Management," it's essential to reflect on the transformative power of embracing a plant-based lifestyle. Beyond the delectable recipes that have graced these pages, this book serves as a gateway to a holistic approach to wellness.

Through the meticulously curated 30-day meal plan and diverse array of breakfasts, lunches, dinners, snacks, desserts, and smoothies, we've laid the foundation for a healthier, more sustainable way of eating. The recipes not only tantalize the taste buds but also address the intricate needs of those aiming for weight loss and managing diabetes.

Each dish is a testament to the vibrant flavors and nourishing benefits that plant-based ingredients offer. From the savory lentil and vegetable stew to the indulgent chocolate avocado mousse, these recipes showcase that health-conscious choices need not sacrifice taste.

Beyond the kitchen, this book encourages a shift in perspective. It's an invitation to view food not merely as sustenance but as a powerful tool for well-being. The journey toward weight loss and diabetes management becomes a celebration of flavors, colors, and textures, making the transition to a plant-based lifestyle not just a choice but a delightful adventure.

Remember, this is not a mere cookbook; it's a guide to a lifestyle that nurtures both body and spirit. As you embark on this culinary expedition, may these recipes be the catalyst for positive change, inspiring you to explore, experiment, and savor the richness of plant-based living. Here's to a healthier, more vibrant you, embracing the journey towards well-being with every delicious, plant-powered bite.